THE
3R METHOD™

RESET. REBALANCE. RECLAIM.

YOUR HORMONES AFTER 35+

A CLINICIAN'S GUIDE TO
NAVIGATING PERIMENOPAUSE, MENOPAUSE &
POSTMENOPAUSE
WITH CONFIDENCE AND CLARITY

BY
DR VANESSA SUSANA STIRZAKER

LOND☉N
BOOK PUBLISHER

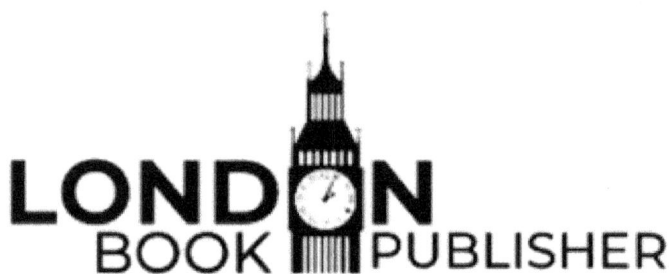

16 East Croft House, 86 Northolt Road,
Harrow, England, HA2 0ER,
United Kingdom

Copyright © 2025 Dr Vanessa Susana Stirzaker

ISBN (978-1-918096-70-5)
ISBN (978-1-918096-71-2)

For more information, visit: www.londonbookpublisher.co.uk

For every woman who was told she was fine when she knew she wasn't. This is for you.

Dedication

To God, the giver of wisdom and strength, may every word of this book bring honour to Your name.

To my late father, Peter Essuah, and my brother, Francis Laud Essuah (RIP, 2024), your absence is felt every day, but your love and legacy live on in me. This book carries your memory forward. To my mother, Rose Yankey, whose faith, love, and sacrifice have carried me further than words can ever express.

To my sister, Belinda Essuah; my sister, Emma; and my brother, William Sam-Aggrey, together with his wife, Iris Angelica Sam-Aggrey, thank you for standing beside me with unwavering belief. To Uncle Douglas Essuah, Uncle Kwame Sam-Aggrey, and Aunt Ruth Yankey, who saw potential in me as a young child and reminded me I could achieve anything I set my heart on.

To my children, Alexander, Simone, and Luna, you are my "why", my joy, and my reason to dream bigger.

And to every woman navigating midlife in the UK, USA, Canada, Europe, Ghana, and beyond, this book is for you. May you find in its pages the strength to Reset, the clarity to Rebalance, and the courage to Reclaim all that is yours.

Dr Vanessa Susana Stirzaker
Founder of Mamichie Healthcare & Creator of the 3R Method™

ACKNOWLEDGEMENTS

To the women whose journeys have inspired every page of this book, thank you. Your courage, resilience, and honesty are the true foundation of this work.

To my mentors, colleagues, and friends: your insights, encouragement, and challenges have sharpened my thinking and enriched my practice. Special thanks to Dr Khalid Mahmood, Consultant Cardiologist, for his behind-the-scenes input and guidance.

To the clinicians, researchers, and global thought leaders whose work is referenced throughout these chapters, thank you for paving the way with your scholarship.

To the women's health communities across the UK, USA, Canada, Europe, Ghana, and beyond, your voices echo in these pages. This mission is bigger than one clinic, one consultation, or one book. It is a call to action for women everywhere.

Finally, to every reader holding this book: thank you for your trust. I hope the 3R Method™ will not only inform you but also guide you to Reset, Rebalance, and Reclaim your health with confidence.

With gratitude and purpose,
Dr Vanessa Susana Stirzaker
Founder of Mamichie Healthcare & Creator of the 3R Method™

TABLE OF CONTENTS

1

You're Not Broken.
You're in Hormonal Transition.

It started with a cup of tea. Not a bad one. Not over-brewed or bitter. Just… unremarkable. I sat across from a woman I'd known for over a decade. Normally bright-eyed, expressive, and full of colour. But that morning? She looked like someone wearing her own face, pale, hollow, flat.

She said, *"I don't even feel like myself anymore. I'm crying at traffic lights. Waking up at 2 a.m. feels like someone's rung an alarm in my brain. I love my kids, but I want to scream by 2 p.m. I've gained a stone, and I swear I haven't changed a thing."*

Then she leaned in with lowered eyes and asked the question I'd heard more times than I could count: *"Am I just going mad… Or is this something else?"*

1.1–The Clinical Truth

This is something else. This is perimenopause. It's not a soft entry into Menopause. It's not "PMS but older." It's not "ageing gracefully". It's a biological shift that impacts your brain, metabolism, mood, memory, immune system, and sense of identity. And it can start in your mid-to-late 30s. No, your periods don't have to stop for it to begin.

Defining Perimenopause, Menopause, and Postmenopause

The conversation around Menopause has been oversimplified for years, reduced to "Your periods stop, and then you're done." That's neither medically accurate nor fair. As a clinician and women's health advocate, I want you to have the real picture: a continuum involving multiple hormones, multiple systems, and decades of life's impact.

Perimenopause—The Hormonal Storm Before the Calm

Perimenopause starts when ovarian activity becomes erratic, often in the late 30s to early 40s. The hormonal changes include:

❖ **Oestrogen fluctuations** (high spikes then sudden crashes) → anxiety, panic, heavy bleeding, and heat intolerance.

❖ **Progesterone decline** → sleep disruption, heightened PMS, and irregular cycles.

❖ **Testosterone gradual decline** → lower energy, libido, and motivation.

❖ **Cortisol hypersensitivity** → exaggerated stress response, fatigue, and insomnia.

❖ **Insulin resistance** → harder weight regulation and metabolic risk.

❖ **DHEA decline** → reduced resilience to stress and less recovery capacity.

❖ **Histamine instability** → migraines, allergies, bloating, and food reactions.

Menopause—The Biological Milestone

Menopause marks the permanent end of ovarian follicular activity, and it's defined by 12 consecutive months without menstruation. The average age is 51.

- ❖ **Oestrogen consistently low** → hot flushes, night sweats, joint stiffness, and urogenital changes.

- ❖ **Progesterone absent** → ongoing sleep and mood fragility.

- ❖ **Testosterone continues declining** → reduced strength, libido, and motivation.

- ❖ **Cortisol & insulin unchecked** → central fat gain and cardiovascular risk.

- ❖ **DHEA diminished** → reduced stress buffering.

- ❖ **Histamine imbalance** → worsening migraines, food sensitivity, and skin changes.

Postmenopause—The Longest Chapter

Postmenopause begins the day after the 12-month mark and continues for the rest of a woman's life. Women may spend one-third to one-half of their lives here.

- ❖ **Oestrogen deficiency** → bone loss, cardiovascular risk, urogenital atrophy.

- ❖ **Progesterone absent** → persistent sleep/mood challenges.

- ❖ **Testosterone deficiency** → loss of muscle, libido, and drive.

- ❖ **Cortisol dysregulation** → immune shifts, fatigue, anxiety.

- ❖ **Insulin resistance** → cardiometabolic disease risk.

- ❖ **DHEA decline** → less resilience.

- ❖ **Histamine imbalance** → persistent inflammation, gut issues, and skin sensitivity.

The 3R Method™ Connection

- ❖ **Reset**: Calm cortisol, stabilise histamine, and protect the brain–gut axis during perimenopause.

- ❖ **Rebalance**: Support hormone integrity and metabolic stability at Menopause.

- ❖ **Reclaim**: Protect bone, brain, and heart health in postmenopause, making this the most empowered chapter of life.

The Hormones

Hormones are not just biochemistry. They are messengers, timekeepers, and translators between your inner and outer world. They decide how you wake in the morning, how your skin feels against your clothes, how steady your moods are in the middle of the day, and how easily you drift into sleep at night. In midlife, these messengers begin to change their rhythm. Understanding them is the first step in Resetting, Rebalancing, and Reclaiming your health.

Oestrogen—The Guardian of Vitality

Definition: Oestrogen is the primary female hormone, produced mainly by the ovaries, with smaller contributions from fat tissue and the adrenal glands.

What it does: It strengthens bone, sharpens memory, balances cholesterol, supports blood vessels, and gives the skin its elasticity.

Progesterone—The Great Stabiliser

Definition: Progesterone is the hormone released after ovulation, designed to balance oestrogen's growth-promoting effects.

What it does: It calms the nervous system, improves sleep quality, reduces anxiety, and prepares the womb for potential pregnancy.

Testosterone—The Spark of Drive

Definition: Testosterone is an androgen, produced in smaller amounts by women's ovaries and adrenal glands.

What it does: It fuels sexual desire, sustains muscle and bone, sharpens focus, and preserves a sense of vitality and drive.

DHEA—The Reservoir Hormone

Definition: Dehydroepiandrosterone (DHEA) is an adrenal hormone that acts as a raw material for both oestrogen and testosterone.

What it does: It supports resilience, mood, and energy, and keeps skin and hair youthful.

Cortisol—The Survival Hormone

Definition: Cortisol is the adrenal hormone released in response to stress, with a natural 24-hour rhythm.

What it does: It regulates blood sugar, blood pressure, immune balance, and how your body copes under pressure.

Thyroid Hormones—The Metabolic Thermostat

Definition: Thyroxine (T4) and triiodothyronine (T3) are iodine-based hormones produced by the thyroid gland.

What it does: They set the body's metabolic pace, influencing heart rate, energy, digestion, and even mood.

FSH—The Brain's Signal to the Ovary

Definition: Follicle-stimulating hormone (FSH) is a pituitary hormone that tells the ovaries to grow eggs and make oestrogen.

What it does: It drives the menstrual cycle by stimulating follicle development.

LH—The Ovulation Trigger

Definition: Luteinising hormone (LH) is a pituitary signal that triggers ovulation and progesterone production.

What it does: It works in tandem with FSH to regulate the cycle.

Prolactin—The Nurturing Hormone

Definition: Prolactin is a pituitary hormone best known for preparing the breasts for milk production.

What it does: Beyond lactation, it influences reproductive balance and immune tone.

Takeaway: These hormones are not abstract. They are the lived forces behind your symptoms. By knowing their language, you gain the clarity to work with your body, not against it. That's where the 3R Method™ begins.

Additional Definitions

To complement the standard definitions of perimenopause, Menopause, and postmenopause, the following terms provide further clinical clarity:

Early Menopause (40–45 years)

Natural Menopause occurs between the ages of 40 and 45, earlier than the population average of ~51 years. Women in this group share many of the same risks as those with POI and premature Menopause, including increased risk of osteoporosis and cardiovascular disease (NICE, 2015; NAMS, 2023).

Premature Menopause (<40 years)

Refers to the permanent cessation of ovarian activity before age 40. This is distinct from Primary Ovarian Insufficiency (POI), where ovarian function may be intermittent. Premature Menopause carries long-term health risks and requires hormone replacement unless contraindicated (ESHRE, 2016).

Induced Menopause

An umbrella term used when Menopause results from medical intervention, typically either surgical Menopause (bilateral oophorectomy) or iatrogenic Menopause (chemotherapy, radiotherapy, or ovarian-damaging surgery).

Types of Menopause

Menopause marks the cessation of ovarian function and menstrual cycles, but its onset, causes, and clinical presentation vary across different types. This section contrasts natural menopause with early menopause, premature menopause, primary ovarian insufficiency (POI), hysterectomy-associated ovarian insufficiency, surgical menopause, and iatrogenic menopause, focusing on their causes, age of onset, symptom patterns, and key management considerations.

Special Cases of Menopause

While the natural transition through perimenopause, Menopause, and postmenopause defines the usual continuum, there are important exceptions where ovarian decline occurs earlier, more abruptly, or as a consequence of surgery or medical treatment. These exceptional cases are critical for clinicians and women alike, as they carry distinct implications for health and management.

Primary Ovarian Insufficiency (POI)

Loss of normal ovarian function before age 40, typically with irregular or absent menses, menopausal-type symptoms, and reduced fertility. Biochemically, oestrogen levels are low with persistently elevated FSH on repeat testing, as outlined by the European Society of Human Reproduction and Embryology (ESHRE, 2016).

Common aetiologies include genetic causes such as Turner mosaicism (Nelson, 2009), FMR1 premutation (ACOG, 2021), autoimmune oophoritis, iatrogenic injury (chemotherapy, pelvic radiation, ovarian surgery), and idiopathic cases.

Clinical implications: Increased long-term risks for bone loss (NAMS, 2023), cardiovascular disease (BMS, 2023), and urogenital atrophy. Physiological hormone replacement is usually recommended until the average age of natural Menopause, unless contraindicated (NICE NG23, 2015). Fertility may be intermittently possible; early fertility counselling/referral should be offered (ESHRE, 2016).

Ovarian Insufficiency After Hysterectomy

When the uterus is removed but the ovaries are left in situ, many women experience menopausal symptoms earlier than expected. This is thought to reflect reduced ovarian blood flow at or after surgery (Farhi et al., 1995), accelerating the decline in ovarian steroidogenesis.

Key points: Cycles cease due to hysterectomy, so the usual marker of Menopause (12 months of amenorrhoea) is unavailable (BMS, 2023). Diagnosis relies on symptoms plus supportive biochemistry, where helpful. Tailored counselling on symptom management and cardiometabolic protection should be provided.

Surgical Menopause

Surgical Menopause refers to the abrupt onset of menopausal symptoms following the removal of both ovaries (bilateral oophorectomy), with or without hysterectomy. Unlike the gradual hormone fluctuations of natural perimenopause, surgical Menopause produces an immediate and profound fall in oestrogen, progesterone, and testosterone (NAMS, 2023).

Clinical picture: More sudden and often more intense vasomotor and neurocognitive symptoms, with rapid loss of the protective effects of ovarian steroids on bone, cardiovascular, urogenital, and metabolic health (BMS, 2023).

Management: In the absence of contraindications, menopausal hormone therapy is generally strongly indicated after premenopausal oophorectomy (NICE NG23, 2015; NAMS, 2023). Address sleep, mood, sexual function, genitourinary symptoms, and long-term bone and heart health; provide psychological support for the dual impact of surgery and hormonal change.

Iatrogenic Menopause

Iatrogenic Menopause occurs when ovarian failure is induced by medical treatment such as chemotherapy, pelvic radiotherapy, or pelvic surgery that damages the ovaries without removing them. The onset may be abrupt or gradual, depending on the agent and dose used (ESHRE, 2016; NAMS, 2023).

Symptoms mirror those of natural and surgical Menopause, but often present earlier and more severely due to the loss of ovarian reserve.

Key considerations include fertility preservation counselling prior to treatment, bone and cardiovascular protection, and early initiation of hormone replacement therapy where appropriate. Psychological support is essential, as women frequently face the dual challenges of cancer survivorship and menopausal transition.

1.2–THE HORMONAL SEESAW OF MIDLIFE

In midlife, ovarian senescence is not a linear decline but a multidimensional, fluctuating system involving endocrine, metabolic, and neuroimmune pathways. Standard texts often reduce this to "low oestrogen," but the lived reality is far more complex. The 3R Method™ framework introduces a new way of mapping these changes—The Hormonal Seesaw—a visual and conceptual model capturing the unstable interplay of hormones, receptors, and feedback loops across midlife.

Key Dynamics at Play:

1. Oestrogen Volatility (Spikes and Troughs)

Sudden surges trigger vasomotor instability, migraines, and anxiety surges. Abrupt troughs dismantle serotonin support, amplifying mood fragility.

2. Progesterone Collapse

Unlike oestrogen's volatility, progesterone demonstrates a progressive, often irreversible collapse, with consequences: disordered sleep, anxiety, and destabilised GABAergic signalling.

3. Androgen Erosion (Testosterone & DHEA Decline)

Slow erosion rather than collapse. Impacts: loss of libido, diminished musculoskeletal integrity, and delayed recovery. Clinically overlooked yet essential for vitality, strength, and repair.

4. Cortisol Hypersensitisation

The HPA axis becomes destabilised, amplifying stress reactivity. What once felt like "normal pressure" now precipitates seismic burnout. Explains why midlife women report disproportionate fatigue in high-stress roles.

5. Metabolic Shift (Insulin Resistance)

Hormonal decline remodels glucose handling and fat distribution. Increased central adiposity and cravings are biological, not moral failings. A precursor to cardiometabolic disease if unaddressed.

6. Histamine and Neuroimmune Crosstalk

Falling oestrogen unmasks histamine hypersensitivity, contributing to migraines, eczema, and bloating. An under-recognised "fourth pathway" linking immunity, hormones, and symptoms of "mystery intolerance."

Why This Matters Clinically?

Standard blood tests report "normal" single-time values, but hormones are dynamic variables, not static markers. The Hormonal Seesaw reframes midlife not as "oestrogen deficiency" but as a multi-axis dysregulation, bridging endocrine, metabolic, neuroimmune, and psychosocial domains. This empowers both women and clinicians to understand why symptoms resist reductionist explanations, and why a personalised, systems-based approach (like the 3R Method™) is required.

1.3–WHY YOU FEEL LIKE YOU'RE LOSING YOURSELF?

Midlife hormonal shifts recalibrate every central system in the body:

❖ **Neurotransmitters** → serotonin and dopamine instability lead to brain fog and mood swings.

❖ **Thermoregulation** → oestrogen withdrawal destabilises the hypothalamus, producing hot flushes and night sweats.

- ❖ **Circadian rhythm** → progesterone loss and cortisol disruption damage sleep architecture, causing insomnia.

- ❖ **Gut–brain axis** → histamine surges and gut permeability trigger bloating, sensitivities, and anxiety.

- ❖ **Self-perception** → testosterone and oestrogen shifts erode confidence, libido, and ambition.

You are not imagining things.

You are not weak.

And you are not broken.

These are measurable biological shifts, not character flaws. Naming them is the first step to reclaiming your power.

1.4–WHAT YOU'VE BEEN MISSING?

What women have been missing is a real framework that integrates science with care. That's why I created the 3R Method™:

- ❖ **Reset** the stress-hormone loop (cortisol, insulin, histamine) so your body stops feeling under siege.

- ❖ **Rebalance** the interconnected systems most affected by midlife hormone shifts, brain, gut, metabolism, immunity, and mood.

- ❖ **Reclaim** your health, clarity, and long-term energy with a personalised plan rooted in both evidence and empathy.

This isn't a passing wellness trend. It's clinical care reimagined for women who've been overlooked for far too long.

1.5–CONCLUSION

If you've ever whispered, "I just don't feel like me anymore," you are not alone. Millions of women across the world echo the same words, often dismissed, often in silence.

This book is your companion through the fog. Together, we'll reset, rebalance, and reclaim. One hand will hold the evidence, hormones, neurotransmitters, and systems medicine. The other will hold real life: your story, your resilience, and your possibility.

You are not broken. You are in transition. With the right map, you will not only find yourself again, but you will also expand into the strongest version of you yet.

2

RESET:
STOP THE CYCLE OF STRUGGLE

For years, I watched women walk into clinic rooms with the same story but different names, different cities, same script:

"I'm exhausted all the time."

"I can't sleep no matter how tired I am."

"I cry at random things and feel numb the rest of the time."

"Every clinician tells me my blood is normal."

One woman clenched her fists as she said, "I keep waiting for this to pass... but it's not passing. It's getting worse."

She wasn't lazy. She wasn't depressed.

She wasn't just busy.

She was over-revved.

Her body was locked in survival mode and didn't know how to come out.

This is where we begin: with the Reset.

2.1–Why Resetting Is the First Step?

Before you can balance hormones, lose weight, or get your joy back, your body needs to feel safe again. Hormones don't shift in isolation. They're deeply tied to your stress response system, primarily the HPA axis (Hypothalamus-Pituitary-Adrenal).

Here's what happens when that system is on overdrive:

❖ Cortisol rises → sleep drops.

❖ Adrenal compensation → anxiety increases.

❖ Blood sugar spikes → cravings + fatigue.

❖ Nervous system overstimulation → brain fog, irritability, and burnout.

If you try to "push through" without a reset, you're pouring energy into a leaking bucket.

2.2–The Clinical Picture of Hormone Stress

This hormonal chaos presents with:

❖ Constant fatigue that doesn't improve with rest.

❖ "Tired but wired" sleep patterns.

❖ Overreacting to minor stressors.

❖ Worsening PMS or irregular periods.

❖ Midsection weight gain despite diet and exercise.

❖ Anxiety is in the body more than in the mind.

Your labs may not flag it, but your life will. This isn't adrenal failure. It's adrenal miscommunication. Your body has been whispering for a while. Now it's yelling.

2.3–WHAT RESET LOOKS LIKE CLINICALLY

A proper reset involves:

❖ Not jumping to HRT without groundwork.

❖ First, calming the nervous system.

❖ Reducing cortisol drivers (blood sugar swings, inflammation, hidden stress).

❖ Restoring circadian rhythm cues (light, movement, protein, rest).

❖ Using targeted nutrition + supplements to support the adrenals and mitochondria.

This is why so many hormone protocols fail: they try to correct the levels before correcting the messaging system.

Why Most Hormone Protocols Fail?—The HRT Conversation

Many hormone replacement protocols fail not because the therapies themselves are ineffective, but because they are delivered into systems unprepared to receive them. Too often, treatment is guided by what appears low on paper, leading to immediate replacement without addressing the underlying regulatory breakdown. Within the 3R Method™, we recognise that stabilisation of the nervous system, circadian rhythm, and cortisol balance is the essential groundwork before any form of hormone therapy can truly succeed.

Hormone Replacement Therapy: Evidence and Application

Contemporary data confirm that breast cancer risk with menopausal hormone therapy (MHT) is dose- and duration-dependent, with higher relative risks for oestrogen-progestogen than for oestrogen-only regimens, and a small excess that wanes after cessation. The 2019 individual-participant meta-analysis from the Collaborative Group provides the largest, most reliable quantification of that pattern. UK-specific, product-level estimates from the 2020 BMJ nested case-control analysis further show heterogeneity between progestogens, with norethisterone conferring the highest and dydrogesterone the lowest relative risks among combined regimens. Randomised WHI follow-up (JAMA 2020) complements these findings: oestrogen-only therapy in hysterectomised women reduced breast cancer incidence and mortality, whereas conjugated oestrogen + MPA increased incidence without affecting mortality. In line with these data, the 2024 NICE update advises that combined HRT modestly increases risk (sequential < continuous), while oestrogen-only has little or no increase; however, NICE deems evidence insufficient to conclude that micronised progesterone or dydrogesterone are definitively safer than other progestogens. The British Menopause Society (2023) cautiously notes observational signals suggesting lower risk with micronised progesterone and dydrogesterone, but emphasises that absolute differences are small and patient-level risk stratification remains paramount.

The Timing Hypothesis

The cardiovascular safety of HRT is strongly influenced by timing. The 'timing hypothesis' suggests that when initiated within 10 years of menopause onset and under the age of 60, HRT carries cardiovascular safety and may even confer benefit (Hodis et al., 2016; Harman et al., 2014). NICE (2024) and the British Menopause

Society (2023) both support this principle, noting higher risks in women who begin HRT later, when vascular ageing and metabolic dysfunction are already established. In cases of premature ovarian insufficiency, replacement is recommended until the average age of Menopause.

Clinical Vignette

A 49-year-old woman presents with persistent vasomotor symptoms and poor sleep. She was started on oral oestrogen by her GP but experienced only partial relief and ongoing insomnia. On review, her cortisol pattern showed evening surges, and her circadian rhythm was disrupted by late-night shift work. After addressing sleep hygiene and introducing strategies to stabilise cortisol, she restarted HRT with transdermal oestrogen and micronised progesterone. This time, symptoms improved significantly and sleep normalised. The difference lay not in the hormones themselves, but in preparing the system to receive them.

Positioning Within the 3R Method™

HRT is not the rescue button it has often been portrayed as. Within the 3R Method™, it is considered a precision instrument to be used after Reset and alongside Rebalance. Prescribing HRT into a dysregulated system is like pouring water into a leaky bucket, temporary improvement without structural repair. Only once the foundation is restored can HRT deliver its full benefit.

2.4–THE MAMICHIE RESET FORMULA™

Inside Mamichie Healthcare, we begin the 3R journey with what I call the Hormone Reset Circuit™, a three-tier framework:

1. Regulate the Nervous System

❖ Breathwork, somatic tools, paced meals, and blood sugar stabilisation.

2. Reset Daily Rhythms

❖ Sleep hygiene, cortisol curve restoration, "sun before screen," light movement.

3. Reduce Hormone Disruptors

❖ Hidden stimulants (too much caffeine, late-night scrolling), gut dysregulation, and inflammatory foods.

This isn't about perfection. It's about giving your body a new baseline, so that when we rebalance? It sticks.

2.5–CONCLUSION

This is the chapter where most women say:

"Why didn't anyone tell me this?"

"Why was I just told to 'take the pill or wait it out'?"

"Why did I blame myself for struggling?"

Because no one ever taught us that a woman's stress response is biologically different. No one told us our midlife hormones are exquisitely sensitive to the world we live in. And so, we blamed ourselves for being tired, heavy, irritable, checked out, and undone.

But the truth is: you don't need to be more resilient. You need a reset.

Reset Action Steps (Toolkit Preview)

These will be expanded in Chapter 10, but here's your first taste:

❖ Start your morning with light + protein.

❖ Stop skipping meals; your blood sugar is not the place to save time.

❖ Replace "I need to push through" with "I'm restoring safety to my system".

❖ Try the 4-7-8 breath technique three times a day.

❖ Take a 10-minute walk after your largest meal to reduce insulin spikes.

Small resets. Big returns.

3

REBALANCE:
FINDING HARMONY IN THE HORMONE STORM

She was in my virtual clinic, sitting in soft morning light, and said something I'll never forget:

"I feel like I'm fighting my own body. Like everything I used to do… just doesn't work anymore. I'm eating 'clean', I'm exercising harder, and somehow, I'm gaining more weight, crying more, and snapping at everyone I love."

She'd seen three specialists.

All her blood tests were "fine." She was told it was "just stress," or worse: "Just your age." But her body wasn't broken. Her body was out of rhythm. And rhythms can be reclaimed. This is the heart of the second "R": Rebalance.

3.1–WHAT HORMONE IMBALANCE REALLY MEANS?

When people hear "hormonal imbalance," they often picture low oestrogen or missing periods. But it's far—deeper and sneakier—than that. Rebalancing is about restoring the functional relationship between multiple systems:

❖ **Oestrogen:** not too low, not too spiky.

- ❖ **Progesterone:** calm, steady, sleep-supportive.

- ❖ **Testosterone:** present, without driving rage or hair loss.

- ❖ **Cortisol:** rising with the sun, easing at night.

- ❖ **Insulin:** sensitive, not screaming.

- ❖ **Thyroid:** supported, not sluggish.

In perimenopause, these systems often swing out of sync, like an orchestra with no conductor. You feel the chaos before you can see it in labs.

Symptoms of Hormonal Disharmony:

Hormonal imbalance is a shapeshifter. It doesn't show up in just one way. It shows up as:

- ❖ Fatigue that defies sleep.

- ❖ Anxiety that feels physical.

- ❖ Rage you don't recognise.

- ❖ Bloating that wasn't there before.

- ❖ Cravings that feel like compulsion.

- ❖ Brain fog mid-conversation.

- ❖ Weight gain without dietary change.

- ❖ Vaginal dryness, low libido, and painful sex.

These are not normal ageing. These are hormonal warning signs.

3.2–HOW WE REBALANCE IN THE 3R METHOD™

Once we've Reset your stress system, we begin the Rebalance Protocol™. This isn't about patching in hormones and hoping for the best. It's about restoring internal harmony with evidence-based, stepwise care.

3.3–THE 5-PILLAR REBALANCE FRAMEWORK

1. **Track the Timeline:** Use symptom patterns, cycle logs, and clinical markers to identify the perimenopause stage. Blood tests are supportive, not definitive.

2. **Feed the Endocrine System:** Prioritise whole proteins, omega-3s, B vitamins, and magnesium. Time meals to support insulin sensitivity + cortisol rhythm.

3. **Support Oestrogen Pathways:** Cruciferous vegetables, fibre, and liver support for safe oestrogen metabolism. Detox isn't a juice cleanse; it's cellular housekeeping.

4. **Restore Progesterone Balance:** Progesterone isn't just about periods; it's your anti-anxiety, pro-sleep hormone. Vitex, magnesium glycinate, and stress recovery practices all play a role.

5. **Review Hormonal Therapy Options:** HRT, bioidentical hormones, topical oestrogen, DHEA, testosterone, all considered with context.

No one-size-fits-all. We assess clinical need, readiness, and safety.

3.4–TESTING, TWEAKING, AND TRUSTING THE PROCESS

Here's what I tell every woman: hormone balance isn't a destination. It's a moving target. You won't always need labs to know you're off; your life is the lab. But when we do test, we look at:

❖ Day 3 and Day 21 hormone panels (if cycling).

❖ Full thyroid panels (not just TSH).

❖ Cortisol patterns (salivary or DUTCH).

❖ Insulin resistance markers.

❖ Inflammatory markers.

Then we tweak with intention, not guesswork, because every woman deserves a treatment plan that's as unique as her story.

What Rebalance Feels Like:

You'll know you've entered the Rebalance zone when:

❖ You wake with energy, not dread.

❖ You can respond, not react, to stress.

❖ Your weight stabilises or shifts without extremes.

❖ You sleep through the night more often than not.

❖ Your libido comes back like an old friend.

❖ You feel like yourself again, maybe even better.

This is not a fantasy. This is your biology… supported correctly.

3.5–CONCLUSION: REBALANCE IN REAL LIFE

It doesn't mean perfection. It represents progress, clarity, and a body that starts to trust you again. You'll have days where things dip. That's okay. Rebalancing is about the long arc of healing, not the perfect week.

In Chapter Four, we'll step into the final R: Reclaimed, where thriving becomes your new normal.

4

RECLAIM:
WHAT THRIVING FEELS LIKE AT MIDLIFE

She was glowing. Not the artificial glow of filters or serums, but the real kind. The kind that says: "I've remembered who I am." She leaned back in her chair and said, "I wake up and don't dread the day anymore. My body feels like a home again, not a battlefield. I'm not snapping at my partner, I'm laughing again. And for the first time in years… I trust myself." This wasn't luck. It wasn't magic. It was the result of a woman who had Reset, Rebalanced, and now finally, Reclaimed.

4.1–THE PURPOSE OF RECLAMATION

Reclaim is about moving from survival to stability, and from stability to thriving. After years of depletion, dysregulation, and dismissal, restoration is a return:

❖ To energy that doesn't fade by 2 p.m.

❖ To mental clarity without caffeine.

❖ To sleep that nourishes, not numbs.

❖ To joy, libido, and ambition that feel natural, not forced.

❖ To hormone health that holds steady, not hostage.

4.2–WHAT RECLAIM MEANS?

Clinically, Reclaiming is the long game. It's what most programmes skip because it's not flashy, but it's where the gold is. Here's what we focus on during the Reclaim phase of the 3R Method™:

1. Mitochondrial Rehab:

Hormones are messengers, but mitochondria are your cellular engines. If they're burnt out, no protocol will work.

Reclaim tools:

❖   CoQ10.

❖   Magnesium.

❖   B vitamins.

❖   Creatine (yes, even for women).

❖   Adaptogens like rhodiola or ashwagandha (if tolerated).

❖   Breathwork + sunlight = mitochondrial signalling.

2. Nervous System Repair:

After years of being in fight-or-flight, you need to live in rest and reclaim.

Reclaim tools:

❖   Cold-to-warm showers (to train vagus nerve response).

❖   Gentle yoga, tai chi, or fascia release.

❖ 10 minutes of stillness daily without a phone.

❖ Safe connection with others (community heals hormones too).

3. Metabolic Strength:

Midlife weight gain is often not just food-related; it's inflammation, insulin, and inactivity driven by fatigue.

Reclaim tools:

❖ Walks after meals.

❖ Strength training 2–3x/week (non-negotiable).

❖ Protein with every meal.

❖ Sleep that improves insulin sensitivity overnight.

❖ Fasting? Only if energy is stable and stress is low.

4. Cycle Awareness or Hormone Replacement Optimisation:

Whether you're still cycling, irregular, or fully postmenopausal, reclaiming is about ongoing awareness.

Reclaim tools:

❖ Seed cycling for still menstruating women.

❖ Regular HRT reviews (dose, delivery method, symptom changes).

❖ Vaginal Oestrogen for sexual wellness and bladder support.

❖ Testosterone for libido, energy, and lean mass (where indicated).

4.3–THE EMOTIONAL SIDE OF RECLAIMING

Let's talk about what no one mentions:

When you start to feel better, it can be scary. You may grieve the years you lost. You may doubt it will last. You may feel guilty for putting yourself first. You may find yourself redefining relationships that thrived on your depletion. This is all part of healing. Reclaiming brings your power back. And with it comes the need to reorganise your life around the woman you've become.

4.4–WHAT THRIVING FEELS LIKE?

It doesn't look like perfection. It looks like peace. Thriving is:

❖ Making decisions from energy, not exhaustion.

❖ Knowing when your hormones are whispering and how to respond.

❖ Enjoying food without fear.

❖ Resting without guilt.

❖ Working from alignment, not urgency.

❖ Feeling confident in your care plan and in your body.

4.5–Conclusion: From Symptom Management to Self-Trust

So many women enter midlife thinking they'll lose who they are. But when you reclaim well, you don't lose yourself, you recover her. The version of you that had been buried under duty, fatigue, and societal silence. This is the "R" that makes the rest worth it.

In the next chapter, we bring the entire 3R Method™ together and demonstrate how it applies in real life through our clinical model, coaching format, and the integrated care plan that supports women worldwide through Mamichie Healthcare.

5

CLINICIAN-BACKED. LIFESTYLE INFORMED. THE 3R MENOPAUSE METHOD™ IN PRACTICE

I didn't set out to build a method. I set out to solve a problem. A smart, successful woman sat in front of me, exhausted, confused, and ashamed, and said, "I went to five different clinicians. I've been told it's stress, my age, depression, and even IBS. But no one has ever looked at my hormones in context." That was the moment I knew: clinical care alone wasn't enough. She didn't need another prescription. She needed a plan. Hence, I created one.

5.1–THE 3R METHOD™ WAS BORN FROM A GAP:

As a clinician, I had seen the gaps in care firsthand:

❖ Hormone therapy is offered without lifestyle support.

❖ Lifestyle advice without medical backing.

❖ "Just wait it out" for perimenopause.

❖ "Here's HRT, see you in a year" for Menopause.

❖ Total neglect of postmenopause care.

The 3R Method™ was born out of the belief that midlife women deserve better, not just symptom relief, but structured recovery and guided transformation.

5.2–WHAT MAKES THE 3R METHOD™ DIFFERENT?

❖ **It's Not a Trend**: It's built on clinical diagnostics, hormone science, lifestyle medicine, and trauma-informed care.

❖ **It's Not a One-Size-Fits-All Plan:** It adapts to whether you're cycling, irregular, postmenopausal, or surgically induced.

❖ **It's Not Either/Or:** You get HRT if it's needed and blood sugar support because it is also needed.

It puts the woman at the centre, not just her symptoms.

5.3–THE CORE CLINICAL PILLARS:

In practice, we assess and address five key systems across all three stages of the 3R Method™:

1. Neuroendocrine Axis, HPA + HPO dysfunction (cortisol, oestrogen, progesterone).

2. Glycaemic Stability, Insulin resistance, cravings, midline weight gain.

3. Thyroid & Mitochondria: Energy metabolism, cold intolerance, fatigue, hair loss.

4. Immune + Inflammatory Response, Autoimmunity, histamine sensitivity, gut disruption.

5. Nervous System + Vagus Nerve Regulation, Anxiety, sleep, overstimulation, vagal tone, trauma memory.

5.4–HOW IT WORKS IN MAMICHIE HEALTHCARE

Whether a woman joins our 1:1 care pathway or group programmes, the structure is always clear:

Step 1: Clinical Case Review: Full symptom timeline, hormonal health history, lifestyle mapping (food, stress, sleep, relationships).

Step 2: Diagnostics + Labs: Hormone panels, thyroid, glucose, cortisol (saliva or DUTCH). Inflammation + gut markers (where needed).

Step 3: Education + Empowerment: We teach her what her body's doing. She learns how to interpret symptoms like data.

Step 4: Her 3R Action Plan™:

❖ **Reset:** Nervous system and adrenal support.

❖ **Rebalance:** Hormone and gut care.

❖ **Reclaim:** Long-term rhythm building, movement, libido, energy.

Step 5: Feedback Loops + Support: Check-ins, progress reviews, symptom tracking. Supplement protocols, HRT (where clinically appropriate). Lifestyle shifts that stick because they're tailored.

The Power of Integration:

We don't throw advice at women and hope it lands. We walk with them. This method has helped:

- ❖ A woman reversed five years of weight gain after early Menopause.

- ❖ A teacher slept through the night again for the first time in a decade.

- ❖ A business owner reignited her libido and reduced hot flushes within weeks.

- ❖ A mum stopped feeling like she was "losing her mind" every cycle.

It works because it sees the whole woman.

5.5–CONCLUSION: THE 3R WAY: WHAT WOMEN SAY

Here's what we hear often:

"I've never had someone explain my body to me this clearly."

"This is the first time I feel seen and not sold to."

"I came for help with hot flushes. I stayed because my entire life feels better."

This is what happens when clinical care and lifestyle support aren't at odds; they're in partnership.

What Comes Next?

In the next chapter, we'll dive into the most misunderstood piece of this journey: Labs vs Symptoms. You'll learn why "normal" labs don't always mean you're well and how to become the expert in your own hormonal story.

6

WHAT LABS WON'T TELL YOU (BUT SYMPTOMS WILL)

She sat down, eyebrows knitted together, holding a thick file.

"All my labs are fine," she said. "Multiple clinicians told me that I'm fine. But I'm not sleeping. I'm snapping at everyone. I can't think straight. And I feel like I'm unravelling."

She passed me the paperwork as if it might unlock a secret. Her oestrogen? In range. TSH? Normal. FSH? Slightly raised. Vitamin D? Borderline. Nothing "alarming." But here's the problem: normal on paper doesn't mean normal in real life.

6.1—THE MYTH OF "NORMAL" LABS

Laboratory ranges are based on population averages, not optimal function. And they rarely account for:

❖ Hormonal fluctuation across the month.

❖ Midlife transitional physiology.

❖ Bio-individual needs.

❖ How do you feel day to day?

Worse still, many standard panels only test TSH (not full thyroid), or single-day oestrogen, or outdated cortisol assays. Women are often told they're "fine" when they're falling apart.

6.2—THE PROBLEM WITH ONE-OFF BLOOD WORK

Hormones are not static. They're rhythmic. Taking one blood sample, without considering:

❖ The day of your cycle.

❖ Your stage of hormonal change.

❖ Your stress level at the time.

It is like taking a photo of a wave and trying to guess the whole tide.

6.3—MOST COMMON MISSED LABS OR MISREAD PANELS

Here's what standard blood tests often miss:

❖ Only TSH is tested for thyroid.

   What's needed: TSH, Free T3, Free T4, Anti-TPO, and sometimes Reverse T3.

❖ Oestradiol is tested randomly.

   What's needed: Day 3 + Day 21 (if cycling) and symptom correlation if not.

❖ Cortisol is tested once in the morning.

   What's needed: Salivary 4-point cortisol or DUTCH test for rhythm.

❖ Insulin not checked.

What's needed: Fasting insulin + HOMA-IR to detect early insulin resistance.

❖ No symptom tracking alongside labs.

What's needed: A clinician who understands what your lived experience is telling them.

6.4—THE SYMPTOM-DRIVEN MODEL

Your hormones speak in signs in the 3R Method™.

We use labs as tools, not dictators. What do we trust more? Your body's report card: symptoms.

❖ Waking at 3 a.m. = possible cortisol imbalance.

❖ Midline weight gain = insulin resistance until proven otherwise.

❖ Cyclical anxiety = likely oestrogen–progesterone imbalance.

❖ Dry eyes, low libido, UTIs = oestrogen deficiency.

❖ Low mood + fatigue + brain fog = screen thyroid and mitochondria.

❖ Rage or tearfulness pre-period = falling progesterone.

These aren't random. They're messages. Symptoms are your body's early warning system.

6.5—How We Use Labs + Symptoms Together

At Mamichie Healthcare, we don't throw out labs, we just put them in context.

We look at:

❖ Your cycle timeline.

❖ Your stress exposure.

❖ Your nutrition, gut health, sleep, and trauma load.

Then we interpret labs like puzzle pieces, not final verdicts.

We track progress by:

❖ Reducing symptom frequency.

❖ Reclaiming daily rhythms.

❖ Watching how you feel, not just how you test.

Why this matters:

Too many women are dismissed because they don't fit the lab-defined illness criteria. But you don't need to be sick to need support. You don't need to be clinically deficient to feel depleted. And you don't need to "wait until it gets worse" to deserve help.

This is the chapter where we rewrite what counts in medicine: your voice, your data, your lived experience.

When symptoms are validated, healing begins.

Once women realise that they're not crazy, not imagining it, not weak, something profound happens:

- ❖ They take charge of their healing.

- ❖ They speak up in medical settings.

- ❖ They seek care that makes sense.

- ❖ They become partners in their plan, not passive recipients.

That's when healing moves from guesswork… to grounded care.

7

YOUR 3R ROADMAP: HOW TO WORK WITH MAMICHIE HEALTHCARE?

By the time most women find us, they're exhausted by options and starving for clarity. They've:

❖ Read 10 different books.

❖ Tried supplements that made things worse.

❖ Felt dismissed in clinical appointments.

❖ Scrolled endlessly on social media for answers.

❖ Wondered if this is just "how midlife has to be."

At Mamichie Healthcare, we offer something different: Not just more information. Not just more products. But a plan that makes sense and supports.

Welcome to your 3R Roadmap.

7.1—WHAT IS THE 3R ROADMAP?

The 3R Roadmap is the structured path we use to guide you through:

1. Reset, calm the chaos, regulate your stress system.

2. Rebalance, address your hormonal, metabolic, and emotional imbalances.

3. Reclaim, build long-term vitality, energy, and confidence.

It is the backbone of every service we offer, whether you're in a 1:1 care plan, a group coaching container, or using our on-demand digital programmes.

7.2—THREE WAYS TO WORK WITH MAMICHIE HEALTHCARE™

1:1 Clinical Care—For You If: you want personalised hormone testing, clinical assessment, and a clinician to walk with you every step of the way. What's included:

❖ Full symptom and hormone timeline.

❖ Bespoke lab testing.

❖ Custom Reset/Rebalance/Reclaim plan.

❖ Supplement + nutrition guidance.

❖ HRT evaluation (if appropriate).

❖ Regular check-ins and support.

❖ WhatsApp/Zoom or email access between sessions.

This is where we go deep. No guesswork. Just grounded, strategic care tailored to your body.

7.3—GROUP PROGRAMS

The 3R Menopause Method™ Circle Is For You If: you want expert guidance, community support, and the structure of a proven framework, without the 1:1 price point.

What's included:

- ❖ 6–12-week group sessions led by Dr Stirzaker.

- ❖ Weekly education modules.

- ❖ Q&A coaching calls.

- ❖ Hormone symptom tracker.

- ❖ Food, mood & cycle templates.

- ❖ Optional lab add-ons.

You're not alone, and this is where you'll prove it to yourself. Community heals. Structure empowers.

Self-Led Programs & Digital Tools—for you if: you're not ready for live sessions but want high-quality, step-by-step resources to get started now.

What's included:

- ❖ On-demand videos.

- ❖ Hormone symptom maps.

- ❖ Reset toolkit.

- ❖ Menopause mini course.

❖ Email series + check-in worksheets.

Affordable, accessible, and immediate. Start today, on your terms.

Our signature tools, every woman in our ecosystem has access to:

❖ The 3R Hormone Symptom Tracker™.

❖ The Reset Your Stress Response Mini-Course.

❖ The Hormonal Nutrition Starter Guide.

❖ The Midlife Lab Review Sheet.

❖ Our private Mamichie Circle forum (for group and 1:1 clients).

These aren't fluffy printables; they're clinically designed, deeply practical tools to help you make sense of what's happening and what's next.

7.4—WHAT HAPPENS WHEN YOU BEGIN?

Here's what to expect, no matter which path you choose:

1. You'll be heard. Your story matters more than your lab numbers.

2. You'll be taught. You'll finally understand why you feel this way.

3. You'll be guided. No generic advice, just clear steps and actual support.

4. You'll begin to feel like you again. Maybe even better.

7.5—CONCLUSION

You're Not Late. You're Right on Time. Many women ask:

"Is it too late for me?"

"What if I've already lost too much ground?"

"What if I've been stuck in this for years?"

Here's what I tell them: your body remembers. Healing is always possible. And midlife isn't the end. It's your Reset. If you're here—reading this—then you're ready. Let's walk the 3R Roadmap together.

8

STORIES OF RESET: CLIENT CASE NARRATIVES

"We don't just treat symptoms. We guide women back to themselves."

—*Dr Vanessa Susana Stirzaker*

Why These Stories Matter?

It's one thing to read about hormones and healing.

It's another to see it unfold, in women just like you. These aren't Instagram quotes or anonymous testimonials.

These are women who walked through exhaustion, confusion, and hormonal chaos, and came out the other side with clarity, confidence, and restored vitality.

Each story you're about to read is used with permission.

Names have been changed.

The triumphs are real.

8.1—CASE 1: AMARA, 44

"I Thought I Was Just Failing at Life."

Symptoms:

❖ Daily anxiety.

❖ Middle-of-the-night wake-ups.

❖ Snapping at her kids.

❖ Deep guilt and shame.

❖ 7 kg weight gain in 8 months.

❖ Periods are still regular.

Background: Amara was a working mother of three. She'd been dismissed by multiple clinicians who said, "It's just stress." Bloods? Normal. Thyroid? Normal. She was even offered antidepressants twice.

3R Intervention: We identified that she was in early perimenopause with significant HPA axis dysfunction. She began a Reset protocol focused on:

❖ Nervous system regulation.

❖ Blood sugar stability.

❖ Magnesium, B-complex, adaptogens.

❖ Sleep window restoration.

By Week 4, her night wakings had reduced. By Week 8, she stopped snapping daily. By Week 12, she had lost 4 kg without focusing on weight.

"I didn't need medication. I needed a map. I needed someone to see me. That's what Mamichie gave me."

8.2—CASE 2: SANDRA, 52

"I Thought It Was Just Menopause."

Symptoms:

❖ Hot flushes.

❖ Vaginal dryness.

❖ Zero libido.

❖ Brain fog.

❖ Fatigue that didn't match her lifestyle.

Background: Sandra was fully menopausal but had avoided HRT out of fear. She'd tried endless supplements with little success. Her marriage was quietly suffering. Her confidence was at an all-time low.

3R Intervention: After a full assessment, we introduced:

❖ Topical vaginal oestrogen.

❖ Transdermal oestrogen + micronised progesterone.

❖ Creatine + omega-3s.

- ❖ A strength-building Reclaim plan.

- ❖ Communication coaching to repair relational strain.

At 3 months, Sandra reported a "return of mental sharpness."

At 5 months, she'd resumed intimacy without pain for the first time in two years.

"I got my body back. I got myself back. And I didn't realise how much I'd missed her."

8.3—CASE 3: LESLEY, 61

"No One Talks About Postmenopause."

Symptoms:

- ❖ Joint stiffness.

- ❖ Urinary urgency.

- ❖ Fatigue.

- ❖ Trouble concentrating.

- ❖ Depression symptoms.

- ❖ Felt "invisible" in healthcare.

Background: Lesley had been told she was "through it." But she didn't feel better, she felt abandoned. Every clinician's visit ended with vague advice or a prescription for statins.

3R Intervention: We focused on postmenopause restoration:

- ❖ Low-dose vaginal oestrogen.

- ❖ Mitochondrial support (CoQ10, magnesium, vitamin D).

- ❖ Pelvic floor therapy.

- ❖ Gentle daily movement (replacing excessive cardio).

- ❖ Gut–brain axis repair (probiotics + dietary shifts).

Lesley regained her spark slowly but surely. She took a solo holiday for the first time in 20 years.

"I didn't know postmenopause could be a chapter. I thought it was just… after. Now I feel stronger at 61 than I did at 45."

8.4—WHAT THESE WOMEN HAVE IN COMMON?

Not their symptoms. Not their supplements. Not even their hormones. What they shared was this: they were dismissed. They were exhausted. And they were done waiting to feel better. When they were given a plan + partnership, they didn't just improve, they transformed.

8.5—CONCLUSION

Reading this chapter, maybe you feel that glimmer:

"Could that be me?"

"Could I finally sleep… stop snapping… feel vibrant again?"

Yes. It can be. And you don't have to do it alone.

9

YOU'RE RIGHT TO ASK FOR MORE

They rolled their eyes. Maybe they said, "It's just your age." "Your labs are fine." "This is what happens to women."

Maybe they told you to meditate. Maybe they prescribed an antidepressant. Maybe they offered the Pill as a catch-all bandage. Maybe they didn't offer anything at all.

You left feeling unheard, unseen, and uncertain if this was all in your head.

Let this be the page that makes it clear: you were right to ask for more.

More answers.

More options.

More respect.

More care.

9.1—YOU WERE RIGHT TO QUESTION THE STANDARD

You were right to wonder:

❖ Why was I never taught this in school?

❖ Why did no one mention that perimenopause could start in my 30s or early 40s?

❖ Why don't we talk about postmenopause as an active hormonal phase?

❖ Why do I feel invisible in clinics, dismissed in consultations, and left to figure it out on Instagram?

This isn't a personal failure. It's a public health oversight. But the tide is turning, and you are part of that shift.

9.2—YOU DON'T NEED TO APOLOGISE FOR WANTING CLARITY

Wanting to sleep well. To think clearly. To stop crying for no reason. To want sex again, or to not feel broken because you don't. These are not "luxuries". They are signals of wellness. Women have been taught to minimise their symptoms and maximise their output. But you were made for more than just pushing through.

9.3—YOU DESERVE A NEW STANDARD OF CARE

A care model that:

❖ Looks at the whole woman.

❖ Listens before prescribing.

❖ Treats your story as clinical data.

❖ Integrates lifestyle with labs.

❖ Treats Menopause not as a dead end, but as a reset button.

That's what we've built at Mamichie Healthcare. That's what you've seen across this book. That's what's waiting for you, whenever you're ready.

9.4—YOUR HORMONES ARE MESSENGERS—NOT VILLAINS

Midlife hormones don't betray you. They reveal you. They force you to slow down, tune in, and re-evaluate. Not because you're weak, but because you're evolving. This is your biology, not your brokenness. And now, you have a way forward.

9.5—YOU WERE ALWAYS WORTH THIS LEVEL OF CARE

Not after your labs showed something. Not after your symptoms got "bad enough". Not after you'd tried everything else. You were worth this from the beginning. And if no one has told you that yet, let this be the moment. You were right to ask for more. And now you have it.

In the final chapter, we leave you with resources, checklists, and tools to carry this forward, whether you work with us, or use this method in your own life starting today.

10

RESOURCES + RESET TOOLKIT

You've made it to the end of this book, but more importantly, you've made it to the beginning of your restoration. Whether you feel ready to dive into your 3R journey or you're simply beginning to understand what's been happening in your body, this chapter is your toolkit. These are the practical steps, clinical insights, and lifestyle rituals that make hormone healing a reality in everyday life. You don't need to do everything at once. You just need to begin.

10.1—THE 3R RESET TOOLKIT™

Step 1: Symptom Tracker—What's Your Hormonal Pattern?

You can't change what you don't track.

Start with our 3R Symptom Tracker™ (available free at MamichieHealthcare.com) and map your:

❖ Sleep quality.

❖ Mood shifts.

❖ Cravings.

❖ Menstrual patterns.

❖ Energy levels.

❖ Libido.

❖ Bloating/inflammation.

❖ Hot flushes/sweats.

Use this for 30 days, and patterns will begin to emerge.

Step 2: The 3R Daily Foundations Checklist

These are the non-negotiables we recommend to every woman in our clinic and coaching programmes. They're simple. They're strategic. And they work.

❖ Water before caffeine.

❖ 30g protein within 90 minutes of waking.

❖ 10+ minutes of daylight exposure by 10 a.m.

❖ Movement after meals (even just 5–10 minutes).

❖ Wind down with light off-screens by 9:30 p.m.

❖ 7–9 hours of sleep, as uninterrupted as possible.

❖ Deep breathing or somatic pause ×3 daily.

❖ Vitamin D/K2 + Magnesium + B-complex (if tolerated).

Step 3: Hormone-Smart Testing (Optional but Recommended)

Here's what we suggest for lab work, especially if you're seeing a clinician:

❖ Day 3 hormones: FSH, LH, Estradiol.

- ❖ Day 21 (or luteal phase): Progesterone.

- ❖ Full thyroid panel: TSH, Free T3, Free T4, Anti-TPO.

- ❖ Fasting insulin + HOMA-IR.

- ❖ Vitamin D3, B12, Ferritin.

- ❖ 4-point salivary cortisol or DUTCH test (advanced).

- ❖ CRP or ESR (inflammation markers).

Bring these to a clinician who understands hormonal transitions, not just fertility or disease.

Step 4: Mindset Reminders for the Healing Process

Hormone healing is not linear. Energy returns in waves. Emotions rise when cortisol lowers. Relationships shift as you reclaim power. Progress is often invisible at first. You're not behind – you're becoming.

Repeat after me:

"I am not broken. I am in transition. And I deserve support through all of it."

10.2—WHERE TO GO FROM HERE?

- ❖ **1:1 Care Pathway:** Book a clinical hormone review with Dr Stirzaker or a Mamichie clinician here.

- ❖ **Group Coaching**: Join our 3R Method™ Circle for evidence-based group care and weekly support.

- ❖ **Self-Led Programmes**: Explore our digital Reset Starter Kits and Hormone Education Library at your own pace.

- ❖ **Stay Connected**: Subscribe to *The Midlife Reset* email list for tools, stories, and science-backed strategies.

10.3—BONUS RESOURCES

- ❖ **Books We Recommend:**
  - ○ *The Menopause Manifesto*–Dr Jen Gunter.
  - ○ *The XX Brain*–Dr Lisa Mosconi.
  - ○ *Glucose Revolution*–Jessie Inchauspé.
  - ○ *This Is Going to Hurt*–Adam Kay (for a laugh).

- ❖ **Podcasts:**
  - ○ *The Doctor's Kitchen.*
  - ○ *Feel Better, Live More.*
  - ○ *On Being* (for nervous system support).

- ❖ **Apps for Midlife Wellness:**
  - ○ Insight Timer (meditation).
  - ○ MyFlo or Clue (cycle tracking).
  - ○ Sleep Cycle (to understand patterns).

10.4—FINAL WORDS FROM DR STIRZAKER

If you've read this far, I want you to hear this: you don't need to hustle your way to healing. You need to Reset, Rebalance, and Reclaim with support.

And when the world tells you you're overreacting, too emotional, or just getting old, you now have the data, language, and tools to say:

"Actually, I'm healing. And I know exactly how."

10.5—THE END AND A BEGINNING

You are not starting over. You are beginning forward. We'll meet you at every step with evidence, empathy, and a method that works.

Welcome to your midlife reset!

THE 3R METHOD™
HORMONE–SYMPTOM ATLAS™

A Clinical Framework for Midlife Symptom Translation

For decades, women have been told that their symptoms are "just stress", "just ageing", or "all in their heads". What has been missing is a clear way to connect the lived experience of symptoms with the biological reality of hormonal change.

The Hormone–Symptom Atlas™ is the first structured tool to:

❖ Map common midlife symptoms directly to their hormonal drivers.

❖ Show the systemic pathways involved, brain, metabolism, immune, cardiovascular, and musculoskeletal.

❖ Provide both women and clinicians with a shared language that validates experience and guides precision care.

Why It Matters?

1. **Symptoms as Signals, Not Failures**—Every hot flush, night sweat, mood swing, or episode of bloating reflects a shift in the body's hormonal ecology.

2. **Beyond Oestrogen**—The Atlas integrates progesterone, testosterone, cortisol, insulin, DHEA, and histamine.

3. **From Story to Strategy**—Move from vague complaints to targeted Reset, Rebalance, and Reclaim strategies.

How to Use This Atlas?

❖ **For women:** Validation—your symptoms are real, explainable, and actionable.

❖ **For clinicians:** Clinical map—link symptoms to biological drivers, guide testing only when useful, and personalise intervention.

❖ **For researchers:** Conceptual framework—a new lens to study Menopause as systemic recalibration, not decline.

INSOMNIA

Symptom	Likely Hormonal Drivers	Systemic Links
Difficulty falling asleep	Low progesterone (↓ GABA)	Brain neurotransmitter imbalance
Waking at 2–3 a.m.	Cortisol surge (circadian disruption)	Adrenal overactivation
Unrefreshing sleep	Low oestrogen (↓ serotonin, melatonin)	Mood & cognition instability
Daytime fatigue	Low testosterone + DHEA	Reduced muscle recovery, immune weakness

ANXIETY

Symptom	Likely Hormonal Drivers	Systemic Links
Sudden panic surges	Oestrogen spikes + histamine release	Neurotransmitter + immune activation
Persistent worry	Low progesterone	Reduced the GABA calming effect
Irritability	Low testosterone	Dopamine imbalance, loss of drive
Racing thoughts	Cortisol excess	Overactive stress response

BLOATING

Symptom	Likely Hormonal Drivers	Systemic Links
Abdominal swelling	Oestrogen fluctuations + histamine	Gut permeability, water retention
Food sensitivities	Histamine instability	Immune overactivation
Constipation	Low progesterone	Reduced gut motility
Gas & cramps	Cortisol stress response	Altered gut microbiome

BRAIN FOG

Symptom	Likely Hormonal Drivers	Systemic Links
Forgetfulness	Low oestrogen ($\downarrow$ acetylcholine)	Cognitive processing decline
Poor concentration	Cortisol dysregulation	Stress-related hippocampal changes
Word-finding difficulty	Low testosterone	Neurotransmitter support loss
Mental fatigue	Low DHEA	Reduced neuroprotection

HOT FLUSHES

Symptom	Likely Hormonal Drivers	Systemic Links
Sudden heat surges	Low oestrogen	Hypothalamic thermostat instability
Night sweats	Oestrogen withdrawal	Thermoregulatory dysfunction
Heart racing with flush	Cortisol + adrenaline surges	Sympathetic overdrive
Drenched sleepwear	Insulin resistance link	Metabolic thermogenesis

JOINT PAIN

Symptom	Likely Hormonal Drivers	Systemic Links
Morning stiffness	Low oestrogen	Cartilage & synovial changes
Widespread aches	Low testosterone	Reduced muscle support for joints
Inflammatory flares	Histamine excess	Immune-related joint pain
Slow recovery after exercise	Low DHEA	Weakened tissue repair

Low Libido

Symptom	Likely Hormonal Drivers	Systemic Links
Loss of sexual desire	Low testosterone	Dopamine drive reduction
Vaginal dryness	Low oestrogen	Urogenital atrophy
Reduced arousal	Low progesterone	Brain calming + intimacy shifts
Exhaustion blocking intimacy	Cortisol excess	Stress prioritises over reproduction

Weight Gain

Symptom	Likely Hormonal Drivers	Systemic Links
Central fat gain	Insulin resistance	Metabolic syndrome risk
Unexplained weight gain despite diet	Low oestrogen	Reduced insulin sensitivity
Loss of muscle mass	Low testosterone	Reduced anabolic drive
Stress-driven eating	Cortisol dysregulation	Reward pathway imbalance

Appendix

A1. THE HORMONAL CONTINUUM (SIMPLIFIED)

Below is the simplified diagram showing oestrogen, progesterone, and testosterone trends across the midlife transition. It is designed for everyday readers to visualise the changes and how the 3R Method™ maps across them.

The Hormonal Continuum of Midlife (Simplified)

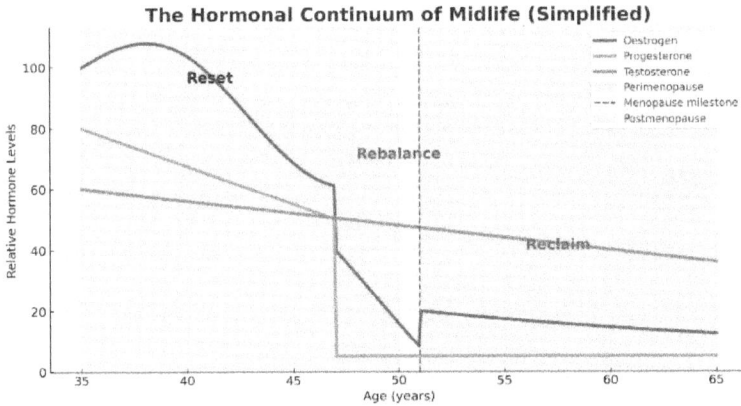

A2. SYMPTOM TRACKER TEMPLATE

Use this tracker monthly to record symptoms and patterns. This helps you see trends and discuss them more effectively with your clinician.

Date	Sleep	Mood	Energy	Bleeding	Hot Flushes	Bloating	Libido	Brain Fog	Joint Pain

A3. QUICK REFERENCE TABLES

What's Normal vs What Needs Attention:

❖ Irregular cycles → normal in perimenopause.

❖ Very heavy bleeding (flooding, clots) → seek medical attention.

❖ Hot flushes → expected.

❖ Palpitations, fainting, or chest pain → seek medical attention.

Symptom-to-Hormone Map:

❖ Anxiety → cortisol, oestrogen fluctuations.

❖ Poor sleep → progesterone decline, cortisol imbalance.

❖ Bloating → histamine instability, gut permeability.

❖ Weight gain (central) → insulin resistance, low oestrogen.

❖ Low libido → testosterone decline.

A4. EVERYDAY 3R REMINDERS

❖ **Reset:** Prioritise stress resilience (sleep hygiene, nervous system resets, gut support).

❖ **Rebalance:** Integrate evidence-based hormone care, nutrition, and activity to stabilise systems.

❖ **Reclaim:** Build strength; protect brain, heart, and bones through long-term strategies.

3R Method™ Clinical Toolkit Tables

This appendix provides evidence-based, practical tables for women navigating perimenopause, Menopause, and postmenopause.

Each table is designed as a quick-reference clinical toolkit to complement the 3R Method™ framework.

EVIDENCE-BASED SUPPLEMENTS IN MIDLIFE HORMONES

Supplement	Typical Dosage Range*	Perimenopause	Menopause	Postmenopause	Benefits (Evidence-Based)	Cautions/Notes
Vitamin D5 + K2	Vit D3: 800–2000 IU daily (higher if deficient); Vit K2: 90–180 mcg daily	✓	✓	✓	Bone health, immune regulation, cardiovascular support	Check baseline Vit D; avoid excess; K2 supports calcium metabolism
Calcium (Diet + Supplements)	1000–1200 mg daily total intake	✓	✓	✓	Reduces fracture risk when combined with Vit D	Prefer dietary sources; excess may ↑ kidney stones
Magnesium (Citrate/Glycinate)	200–400 mg daily	✓	✓	✓	Supports sleep, anxiety, muscle relaxation	High doses may cause diarrhea; adjust form
Omega-3 (EPA/DHA)	1–2 g daily	✓	✓	✓	Cardiovascular protection, reduces inflammation, may support mood	Use high-quality fish oil or algae-based for vegetarians
B-Complex (B6, B12, Folate)	Varies (B12 500–1000 mcg daily if deficient)	✓	✓	✓	Energy metabolism, cognition, reduces homocysteine	Monitor B12 in vegans/vegetarians
Phytoestrogens (Soy Isoflavones, Flaxseed)	40–80 mg/day isoflavones	✓	✓	Limited	Modest effect on hot flushes, bone density	Avoid in estrogen-sensitive cancers unless cleared
Probiotics	1–10 billion CFU daily	✓	✓	✓	Supports gut microbiome, estrogen metabolism, immunity	Strain-specific effects; evidence still evolving
Ashwagandha (Adaptogen)	300–600 mg extract daily	✓	✓	✓	May reduce stress/cortisol, improve sleep	Avoid in hyperthyroidism or pregnancy
Rhodiola Rosea	200–400 mg daily	✓	✓	✓	Energy, mood resilience, fatigue	May interact with SSRIs or BP meds
DHEA (Clinical Use Only)	25–50 mg daily	Limited	✓	✓	Improves libido, bone density, mood (when deficient)	Prescription only; monitor androgens/testosterone
Creatine Monohydrate	3–5 g daily (maintenance); 0.1 g/kg body weight daily	✓	✓	✓	Supports muscle strength, bone density, and cognitive performance when combined with resistance training; may reduce fatigue and improve energy metabolism during estrogen decline	Ensure adequate hydration; may cause mild water retention or bloating; avoid in renal impairment or if serum creatinine is elevated; best used with regular exercise

*Dosages are general ranges for adults; individualisation and clinical monitoring are essential.

EVIDENCE-BASED EXERCISE BY HORMONE STAGE

Exercise Type	Frequency & Duration	Perimenopause	Menopause	Postmenopause	Key Benefits	Clinical Notes
Resistance / Strength Training	2–3x/week, 30–45 min	✓	✓	✓	Preserves lean muscle, bone density, boosts metabolism	Focus on progressive load, prevent sarcopenia
Weight-Bearing Cardio	150 min/week moderate OR 75 min/week vigorous	✓	✓	✓	Supports bone strength, cardiovascular health, weight control	Encourage joint-friendly options if arthritis present
HIIT	1–2x/week, 15–20 min	✓	✓	Limited	Improves insulin sensitivity, fat metabolism, VO2 max	Tailor intensity, caution in cardiac risk
Yoga / Pilates	2–3x/week, 20–40 min	✓	✓	✓	Reduces cortisol, improves flexibility, pelvic floor	Strong evidence for stress/anxiety reduction
Balance & Functional Training	2–3x/week, 10–20 min	✓	✓	✓	Fall prevention, coordination, independence	Especially important post-60 yrs
Swimming / Cycling	1–2x/week, 30 min	✓	✓	✓	Cardiovascular fitness without joint strain	Not bone-building, pair with resistance
Pelvic Floor Exercises	Daily, 5–10 min	✓	✓	✓	Prevents incontinence, supports sexual health	Early incorporation = long-term benefit

Nutrition & Global Foods for Hormonal Balance

Nutrient Focus	UK / Europe Foods	US / Canada Foods	Ghana / West Africa Foods	Asia Foods	Benefits in Midlife	Clinical Notes
Protein	Eggs, Greek yogurt, salmon, chicken	Turkey, cottage cheese, whey protein	Tilapia, beans, groundnuts, goat meat	Tofu, tempeh, lentils, fish	Preserves muscle, metabolism, satiety	Aim 1.2–1.6 g/kg/day, distribute across meals
Calcium	Milk, cheese, sardines, fortified plant milks	Dairy, kale, fortified juices	Dried fish, kontomire, millet	Soy milk, bok choy, sesame seeds	Bone health, fracture prevention	Needs Vit D + K2 for absorption
Phytoestrogens	Flaxseed, chickpeas, oats	Soy milk, edamame, lentils	Groundnuts, bambara beans, sorghum	Soybeans, miso, red clover tea	Modest relief of hot flushes, bone density	Best evidence with soy isoflavones 40–80 mg/day
Omega-3	Mackerel, herring, walnuts	Salmon, chia seeds, fish oil	Sardines, anchovies, egusi seeds	Oily fish, seaweed, flaxseed	Mood, cardiovascular, anti-inflammatory	Plant ALA less potent than EPA/DHA
Magnesium	Pumpkin seeds, spinach, dark chocolate	Almonds, avocados, quinoa	Beans, groundnuts, leafy greens	Brown rice, mung beans, sesame seeds	Sleep, anxiety, muscle relaxation	Prefer glycinate/citrate if supplementing
Iron	Red meat, fortified cereals	Beef, spinach, chicken liver	Goat meat, beans, kontomire	Tofu, black beans, dried shrimp	Prevents anemia, fatigue	Avoid excess post-menopause unless deficient
Fiber	Oats, barley, berries	Apples, beans, whole grains	Plantain, cassava, beans	Brown rice, sweet potato, mung beans	Gut health, estrogen metabolism	Aim ≥25–30 g/day
Antioxidants	Berries, olive oil, herbs	Blueberries, cranberries, green tea	Hibiscus tea, baobab fruit, okra	Green tea, turmeric, ginger	Reduces oxidative stress, cardiovascular protection	Prefer food sources over supplements

Red Flag Clinical Symptoms

Symptom	Possible Concern	Action Needed
Heavy bleeding post-menopause	Endometrial pathology (e.g., cancer, hyperplasia)	Urgent gynaecology referral
New severe headaches + visual changes	Neurological disorder (tumour, raised ICP)	Neurology review
Unexplained weight loss >5%	Malignancy, thyroid disease	Full clinical workup
Persistent bloating/abdominal pain	Ovarian or GI cancer	Ultrasound + urgent referral
Chest pain or exertional breathlessness	Cardiac disease, pulmonary embolism	Emergency evaluation
Unilateral leg swelling/pain	DVT	Immediate vascular/ED assessment

Hormone Replacement Therapy (HRT) Reference Table

Hormone	Typical Preparations & Doses	Perimenopause	Menopause	Postmenopause	Key Notes
Estrogen	Patch: 25–100 mcg/day Gel: 1–4 pumps (0.75–3 mg) Oral: 1–2 mg/day	✓ (cyclic w/ progesterone)	✓ (cyclic or continuous)	✓ (often lower dose)	Transdermal preferred for VTE risk; oral ↑ clot/stroke risk
Progesterone (micronised)	100 mg daily continuous 200 mg x 12–14 days/month	✓ (if uterus present)	✓	✓ (continuous often used)	Protects endometrium if uterus intact
Combined HRT	Oral or patch	✓	✓	✓	Convenient, less flexible for dose adjustment
Testosterone (specialist)	300 mcg/day gel/cream	Limited	✓ (low libido, HSDD)	✓	Specialist prescribing only, monitor levels
DHEA (Intrarosa®)	6.5 mg vaginal pessary daily	—	✓ (for GSM atrophy)	✓	Good for vulvovaginal atrophy when systemic HRT not suitable

⚠ This table is based on guidance from NICE (UK), the British Menopause Society (BMS), and the North American Menopause Society (NAMS). It is intended as a discussion tool for healthcare providers, not for self-medication or self-prescription. Individualised treatment and monitoring are essential.

Life Stage Priority Table (40s vs 50s vs 60s+)

Age Group	Hormone Priorities	Lifestyle Priorities	Clinical Checks
40–49 (Perimenopause)	Estrogen fluctuations, progesterone decline, cortisol dysregulation	Sleep hygiene, stress reduction, exercise habits, fertility awareness	FSH/LH (contextual), thyroid screen, Vit D, iron/ferritin, lipid baseline
50–59 (Menopause transition)	Estrogen deficiency, ↑ bone turnover, metabolic changes	Resistance training, heart health, bone + muscle nutrition, weight control	Bone density scan (if risk), HbA1c, lipids, BP, cervical/breast screening
60+ (Postmenopause)	Low estrogen, ↓ androgens, sarcopenia risk	Fall prevention, joint protection, functional training, nutrition for longevity	Bone density, cardiac screen, diabetes risk, memory/cognitive baseline

GLOBAL MENOPAUSE TIMELINE TABLE

Region	Avg Age at Menopause	Cultural Practices	Diet Patterns
UK / Europe	51 yrs	HRT widely available; awareness campaigns	Dairy, fish, greens, Mediterranean
North America	51–52 yrs	High HRT uptake in some states; advocacy groups	High protein, fortified foods, supplements
West Africa	48–49 yrs	Herbal medicine, community-led care	Millet, plantain, beans, fish, groundnuts
Asia	49–50 yrs	Lower vasomotor symptoms; soy-rich diets	Soy, tofu, miso, rice, green tea
Latin America	46–48 yrs	Family/community support; less HRT uptake	Beans, corn, rice, tropical fruits

MEDICATION & NON-HRT OPTIONS TABLE

Category	Example	Symptom Targets	Evidence Strength	Key Notes
SSRIs/SNRIs	Venlafaxine, Paroxetine, Escitalopram	Hot flushes, mood	Moderate (NAMS/NICE approved)	Low-dose effective; avoid abrupt withdrawal
Gabapentin	300–900 mg/day	Hot flushes, sleep	Moderate	Sedating; useful at night; dizziness possible
Clonidine	25–50 mcg BID	Hot flushes	Low–moderate	Often poorly tolerated (dry mouth, hypotension)
Vaginal Estrogen	Estriol/Estradiol pessaries, creams, rings	Vaginal dryness, GSM	Strong	Safe long-term; minimal systemic absorption
Herbal / Botanicals	Black cohosh, Red clover, Sage	Hot flushes, mood, sleep	Variable/weak	Mixed evidence; liver caution (black cohosh)
Lifestyle Medicine	CBT, yoga, paced breathing	Insomnia, hot flushes, anxiety	Strong for CBT; moderate for yoga	Safe, scalable, good adjunct to HRT

Clinician Key Takeaways: The Hormonal Seesaw

The Hormonal Balance™ of Midlife

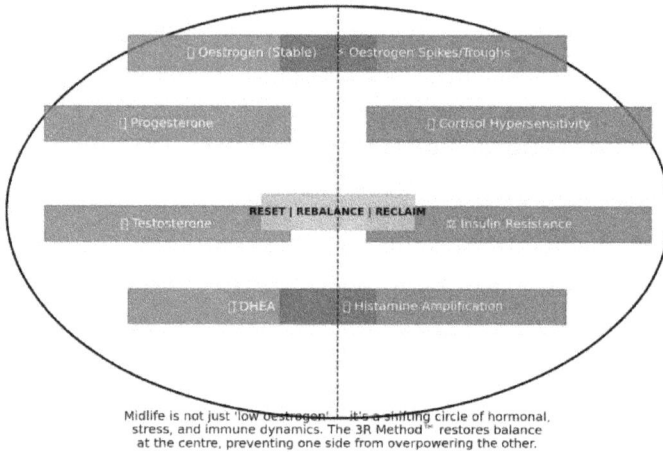

Oestrogen (Stable)	Oestrogen Spikes/Troughs
Progesterone	Cortisol Hypersensitivity
Testosterone	RESET | REBALANCE | RECLAIM	Insulin Resistance
DHEA	Histamine Amplification

Midlife is not just 'low oestrogen'—it's a shifting circle of hormonal, stress, and immune dynamics. The 3R Method™ restores balance at the centre, preventing one side from overpowering the other.

This insert provides a concise, practice-oriented synthesis of the Hormonal Seesaw model, highlighting its clinical implications for midlife care.

Midlife instability is multidimensional.

Do not reduce symptoms to "low oestrogen." The seesaw model recognises fluctuations across multiple axes: endocrine, metabolic, and neuroimmune.

Hormones are dynamic, not static.

Single-time blood tests can miss the reality of hourly fluctuations. Clinical interpretation requires context, symptom mapping, and sometimes sequential testing.

Progesterone collapse precedes oestrogen deficiency.

Disrupted GABA signalling explains early insomnia and anxiety, often misattributed to psychiatric causes.

Androgen decline is clinically significant.

Testosterone and DHEA are critical for libido, musculoskeletal integrity, and resilience. Their erosion is under-recognised in routine care.

Cortisol hypersensitivity drives burnout.

Heightened HPA reactivity explains disproportionate stress fatigue in high-functioning midlife women.

Metabolic and immune crosstalk.

Insulin resistance and histamine sensitivity amplify weight, cravings, migraines, and gut-skin symptoms, areas often overlooked in consultations.

Systems-based management is essential.

Personalised, integrative strategies—like the 3R Method™—are better suited to restoring balance than one-size-fits-all hormone prescriptions.

The Hormonal Seesaw: What It Means for You

Midlife hormones don't simply 'run out', they shift, spike, and fall in ways that can feel confusing. The Hormonal Seesaw helps explain why you may feel fine one week and completely different the next. It shows that your symptoms are real, biological, and part of a bigger pattern, not your fault.

The Hormonal Seesaw™ of Midlife

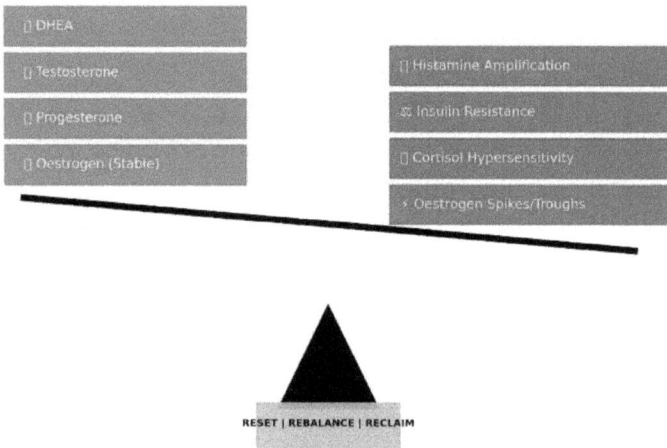

DHEA

Testosterone

Progesterone

Oestrogen (Stable)

Histamine Amplification

Insulin Resistance

Cortisol Hypersensitivity

Oestrogen Spikes/Troughs

RESET | REBALANCE | RECLAIM

Midlife is not just 'low oestrogen' — it's a shifting seesaw of hormones, stress pathways, and immune signals. The 3R Method™ restores balance by Resetting, Rebalancing, and Reclaiming this system.

Oestrogen ups and downs

Can feel like sudden hot flushes, heavy periods, or migraines.

Progesterone drop

Often, the reason for poor sleep, anxiety, and mood swings.

Testosterone and DHEA decline

Energy, sex drive, and recovery after exercise can feel harder to maintain.

Stress hormones on overdrive

Small pressures can suddenly feel overwhelming, leading to burnout or crashes.

Metabolism shifts

Weight can be harder to shift, cravings increase, and belly fat appears even without major lifestyle changes.

Histamine sensitivity

Bloating, itchy skin, or migraines may flare when hormones dip.

The key message: your symptoms are not random or imagined, they are signals from your body. With the right support and a personalised plan, balance can be restored.

Professional Resources

P1. THE HORMONAL CONTINUUM (CLINICAL VERSION)

This version includes oestrogen, progesterone, testosterone, cortisol, insulin, DHEA, and histamine trends. It illustrates the multi-system interplay of the midlife transition.

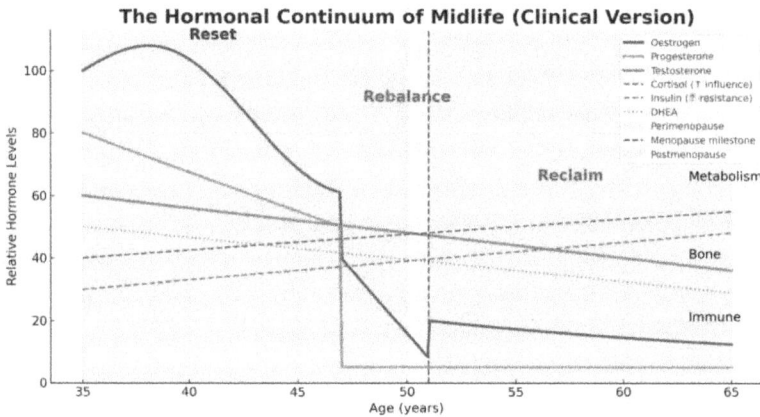

The Hormonal Continuum of Midlife (Clinical Version)

P2. 3R METHOD™ CLINICAL FRAMEWORK

❖ **RESET** → Assess and address cortisol, insulin resistance, and histamine response.

❖ **REBALANCE** → Precision hormone replacement (oestrogen, progesterone, testosterone) and lifestyle stabilisation.

❖ **RECLAIM** → Long-term monitoring and protection of bone, brain, cardiovascular, and immune health.

P3. HORMONAL BIOMARKERS

Key markers for evaluation:
* ❖ FSH, LH, Oestradiol, Progesterone.

* ❖ Free Testosterone, SHBG.

* ❖ DHEA-S, Cortisol.

* ❖ Insulin, fasting glucose, HbA1c.

* ❖ CRP, inflammatory markers.

* ❖ Histamine (clinical suspicion + gut testing).

P4. GLOBAL CLINICAL GUIDELINES

Comparison of leading menopause society guidelines:

* ❖ UK NICE → Emphasis on shared decision-making, HRT is safe for the majority.

* ❖ North American Menopause Society (NAMS) → Strong support for body-identical HRT as first-line.

* ❖ European Menopause and Andropause Society (EMAS) → Focus on early intervention, cardiovascular and bone protection.

These converge on one message: body-identical hormone therapy, lifestyle medicine, and personalised care are safe and effective.

Master Bibliography – The 3R Method™ Book

❖ American College of Obstetricians and Gynaecologists (ACOG). (2017). Practice Bulletin No. 141: Management of menopausal symptoms. *Obstetrics & Gynaecology*, 126(1), 1–21.

❖ American College of Obstetricians and Gynaecologists (ACOG). (2021). Primary ovarian insufficiency. ACOG Practice Bulletin No. 223. *Obstetrics & Gynaecology*, 137(6), e138–e152.

❖ Avis, N.E., Crawford, S.L., & Greendale, G.A. (2022). Midlife health in women: Menopause transition and ageing. *Lancet*, 399(10334), 1243–1256.

❖ Baber, R.J., Panay, N., Fenton, A., & IMS Writing Group. (2016). 2016 IMS Recommendations on women's midlife health and menopause hormone therapy. *Climacteric*, 19(2), 109–150.

❖ Balachandran, D.D., Faiz, S.A., & Jasper, N.R. (2021). Sleep and Menopause: Associations with vasomotor symptoms, mood, and health outcomes. *Sleep Medicine Reviews*, 55, 101381.

❖ British Menopause Society (2022). Tools for clinicians: Hormone Replacement Therapy guidance.

- British Menopause Society (BMS). (2023). BMS Consensus Statement: Hormone replacement therapy and alternatives for the management of menopausal symptoms. London: BMS.

- British Menopause Society (BMS). (2023). Consensus statement: Management of the Menopause. *Post Reproductive Health*, 29(2), 63–82.

- British Menopause Society. (2023). BMS & WHC's recommendations on HRT in menopausal women (Sept 2023 update). Stratford-upon-Avon: BMS.

- Burger, H.G., Hale, G.E., Robertson, D.M., & Dennerstein, L. (2007). A review of hormonal changes during the menopausal transition: Focus on findings from the Melbourne Women's Midlife Health Project. *Human Reproduction Update*, 13(6), 559–565.

- Chlebowski, R.T., Aragaki, A.K., Anderson, G.L., Manson, J.E., Stefanick, M.L., Pan, K., Barrington, W., Kuller, L.H., Simon, M.S., and Lane, D.S. (2020). Association of menopausal hormone therapy with breast cancer incidence and mortality during long-term follow-up of the Women's Health Initiative randomised clinical trials. *JAMA*, 324(4), pp.369–380.

- Collaborative Group on Hormonal Factors in Breast Cancer, 2019. Type and timing of menopausal hormone therapy and breast cancer risk: individual participant meta-analysis of the worldwide epidemiological evidence. *The Lancet*, 394(10204), pp.1159–1168.

- Epel, E.S., Crosswell, A.D., Mayer, S.E., et al. (2018). More than a feeling: A unified view of stress measurement for population science. *Frontiers in Neuroendocrinology*, 49, 146–169.

❖ European Society of Human Reproduction and Embryology (ESHRE). (2016). ESHRE Guideline: Management of women with premature ovarian insufficiency. *Human Reproduction*, 31(5), 926–937.

❖ ESHRE (European Society of Human Reproduction and Embryology), 2016. ESHRE Guideline: Management of women with premature ovarian insufficiency. Brussels: ESHRE. Available at: Guideline on premature ovarian insufficiency [Accessed 12 September 2025].

❖ Farhi, J., Ben-Haroush, A., & Lunenfeld, B. (1995). Ovarian function following hysterectomy with ovarian conservation: A review. *International Journal of Fertility*, 40(2), 76–81.

❖ Freeman, E.W., Sammel, M.D., & Lin, H. (2020). Temporal associations of hot flushes and depression in the transition to Menopause. *Menopause*, 27(1), 1–7.

❖ Gordon, J.L., Rubinow, D.R., & Eisenlohr-Moul, T.A. (2019). Hormone variability and mental health in perimenopause: A review of recent evidence. *Current Psychiatry Reports*, 21(7), 57.

❖ Heiss, G., Wallace, R., Anderson, G.L., et al. (2008). Health risks and benefits 3 years after stopping randomised treatment with oestrogen and progestin. *JAMA*, 299(9), 1036–1045.

❖ Jacka, F.N., O'Neil, A., Opie, R., et al. (2017). A randomised controlled trial of dietary improvement for adults with major depression (the 'SMILES' trial). *BMC Medicine*, 15, 23.

❖ Kaunitz, A.M., & Manson, J.E. (2015). Management of menopausal symptoms. *Obstetrics & Gynaecology*, 126(4), 859–876.

❖ Lundell, C., et al. (2024). Breast and endometrial safety of micronised progesterone versus synthetic progestins in MHT: study protocol for a double-blind RCT. *BMJ Open*, 14:e082749.

❖ Manson, J.E., Chlebowski, R.T., Stefanick, M.L., et al. (2013). Menopausal hormone therapy and health outcomes during the intervention and extended post-stopping phases of the Women's Health Initiative randomised trials. *JAMA*, 310(13), 1353–1368.

❖ Manson JE, Kaunitz AM. (2016). Menopause Management— Getting Clinical Care Back on Track. N Engl J Med, 374: 803–806.

❖ Matthews, K.A., & Bromberger, J.T. (2022). Lifestyle influences on midlife women's health: Stress, sleep, and diet. *Annual Review of Public Health*, 43, 199–218.

❖ National Institute for Health and Care Excellence (NICE). (2015). Menopause: Diagnosis and management (NG23). London: NICE.

❖ NICE (2019). Menopause: diagnosis and management. National Institute for Health and Care Excellence Guideline [NG23].

❖ National Institute for Health and Care Excellence (NICE). (2023). Menopause: Diagnosis and management (NG23). London: NICE.

❖ National Institute for Health and Care Excellence (NICE). (2024). Menopause: identification and management. NICE Guideline [NG23]. London: NICE.

❖ Nelson, L.M. (2009). Clinical practice: Primary ovarian insufficiency. *New England Journal of Medicine*, 360(6), 606–614.

❖ North American Menopause Society (NAMS). (2022). The 2022 hormone therapy position statement of The North American Menopause Society. *Menopause*, 29(7), 767–794.

❖ North American Menopause Society (NAMS). (2023). The 2023 position statement: Hormone therapy and other management of menopause-related symptoms. *Menopause*, 30(7), 678–708.

❖ North American Menopause Society (2023). The 2023 Nonhormone Therapy Position Statement.

❖ Phillips, D.I.W., Barker, D.J.P., Fall, C.H.D., et al. (2000). Elevated plasma cortisol concentrations: A link between low birthweight and insulin resistance syndrome? *Journal of Clinical Endocrinology & Metabolism*, 85(7), 2676–2678.

❖ Santoro, N., & Randolph, J.F. (2011). Reproductive hormones and the menopause transition. *Obstetrics & Gynaecology Clinics of North America*, 38(3), 455–466.

❖ Santoro N, Epperson CN, Mathews SB. (2015). Menopausal Symptoms and Their Management. Endocrinology and Metabolism Clinics of North America, 44(3): 497–515.

❖ Sowers, M., Zheng, H., Tomey, K., et al. (2007). Changes in body composition in women over six years at midlife: The Study of Women's Health Across the Nation. *American Journal of Medicine*, 120(10), e1–e8.

❖ Sourouni, M., Ortmann, O., & Treeck, O. (2023). Menopausal hormone therapy and the breast: a review. *Breast Care*, 18(3), 164–175.

❖ Stuenkel, C.A., Davis, S.R., Gompel, A., et al. (2015). Treatment of symptoms of the Menopause: An Endocrine Society clinical practice guideline. *Journal of Clinical Endocrinology & Metabolism*, 100(11), 3975–4011.

❖ Thurston, R.C., & Joffe, H. (2011). Vasomotor symptoms and menopause: Findings from the Study of Women's Health Across the Nation. *Obstetrics & Gynaecology Clinics*, 38(3), 489–501.

❖ Thurston, R. et al. (2020). Vasomotor symptoms: physiology, risk factors, and relation to cardiovascular disease. Menopause, 27(7), 723–731.

❖ U.S. Preventive Services Task Force (USPSTF). (2017). Hormone therapy for the primary prevention of chronic conditions in postmenopausal women: USPSTF recommendation statement. *JAMA*, 318(22), 2224–2233.

❖ Vedhara, K., Hyde, J., Gilchrist, I.D., et al. (2000). Acute stress, memory, attention and cortisol. *Psychoneuroendocrinology*, 25(6), 535–549.

❖ Warren, M.P., & Halpert, S. (2020). Hormone therapy in midlife women: Clinical applications. *Endocrinology and Metabolism Clinics of North America*, 49(4), 517–534.

❖ Westerterp-Plantenga, M.S. (2016). Nutrition and hormones in the regulation of energy metabolism: Evidence for the role of ghrelin, leptin, and cortisol. *Nutrition Research Reviews*, 29(1), 35–48.

❖ World Health Organisation (WHO). (2021). Women's health and ageing: Global health estimates and policy guidance. Geneva: WHO.

❖ Vinogradova, Y., Coupland, C., & Hippisley-Cox, J. (2020). Use of hormone replacement therapy and risk of breast cancer: nested case-control studies using the QResearch and CPRD databases. *BMJ*, 371, m3873.

ABOUT THE AUTHOR

Across the world, women over 35 are too often dismissed when their hormones begin to shift. They're told to *cope*, to *get on with it*, or worse, that it's *all in their heads*. The truth is: midlife isn't a time of decline, it's a time of potential. I believe every woman deserves to thrive, not just survive, through perimenopause, Menopause, and beyond.

This belief inspired me to develop the 3R Method™: Reset, Rebalance, Reclaim. It's an evidence-based approach that combines the precision of medicine with the practicality of lifestyle tools. My work is rooted in clinical expertise but designed for real life, helping women restore their hormonal integrity, reclaim their energy, and embrace midlife as a season of growth.

I'm Dr Vanessa Susana Stirzaker, clinician, creator of the 3R Method™, founder of Mamichie Healthcare, and global menopause specialist. Over the years, I've supported women from all walks of life to reset their health and reclaim their power. This book is my manifesto, my clinical guide, and my promise: that midlife can be the most empowered chapter yet.

Discover more at www.mamichiehealthcare.com
Instagram: @mamichie_healthcare
Facebook: @mamichiehealthcare

www.ingramcontent.com/pod-product-compliance
Lightning Source LLC
Chambersburg PA
CBHW051248020426
42333CB00025B/3114